DASH DIET COOKBOOK FOR BEGINNERS

THE BLOOD PRESSURE AND WEIGHT LOSS SOLUTION ACTION PLAN COOKBOOK

Table of Contents

Introduction

Of all the 38 healthy diet plans nowadays, the DASH diet has been recognized as the best diet plan for a healthy living lifestyle. It is also recommended for controlling diabetes and contributing to good heart health.
It can be adopted by both vegetarians and non-vegetarians and offers flexibility to meet meal preferences.

DASH: Dietary Approaches to Stop Hypertension

DASH dieting is simply taking care to identify food-based strategies to reduce blood pressure.
It contains a sequence of instructions that an individual has to follow to enjoy all the benefits that this diet plan proposes. To ensure that one attains the goals set for oneself, several factors must be considered, such as:

- Hard work in terms of sticking to the diet plan is required to achieve favorable results

- Self-discipline must be exercised to ensure the timely intake of meals

- It helps to use reminders as well as alarms to keep tabs on progress

- Daily instructions must be religiously followed, depending on individual the eating plans

The DASH diet emphasizes the consumption of fruits (to increase fiber intake and produce sufficient energy), whole grains (excellent sources of fiber and nutrients), dairy products (sources of Vitamin D, calcium and protein), vegetables (for magnesium, fiber, vitamins and potassium), nuts and seeds (contain saturated fat, protein, phytochemicals), and fish and meat (for zinc, iron, protein). The DASH diet can be as effective as medications when it comes to regulation of blood pressure and cholesterol. The lower the intake of sodium, the lower the blood pressure. The DASH diet also restricts consumption of fat (meats, dairy), sugar, sugar-based beverages, sweets and salt. Although the DASH diet is not as effective as low carbohydrates diets in terms of losing weight, if an individual follows this diet plan to the T and adds an exercise routine, he can lose weight and improve both metabolism and sensitivity to insulin.

Recipes

Breakfast

Preparation Time: 15 minutes

Cooking Time: 20 minutes

Serving: 6

Ingredient:

2 cups whole-wheat flour

1 tablespoon baking powder

1½ teaspoons pumpkin pie spice

½ teaspoon kosher or sea salt

2 tablespoons dark brown sugar

4 tablespoons canola oil

2 large eggs

1 cup sweet potato purée or cooked mashed sweet potato

1½ cups nonfat milk

1 teaspoon pure vanilla extract

Cooking spray

1½ cups plain nonfat Greek yogurt

½ teaspoon maple extract or 1 tablespoon pure maple syrup

Direction

Scourge flour, baking powder, pumpkin pie spice, and salt until combined.

Using a separate mixing bowl, with a hand mixer set on medium speed to beat the brown sugar and canola oil together until fluffy. While the hand mixer is still beating, add one egg at a time until thoroughly combined. Add the sweet potato purée then the milk and vanilla extract until well blended. With a hand mixer to low speed and slowly add the dry ingredient mixture until well blended.

Heat a large nonstick skillet over medium heat. Coat the pan with the cooking spray. Working in batches, ladle ¼-cup dollops of pancake batter into the pan. Cook for 1 to 2 minutes, until bubbles appear on the top, then flip and cook for another 1 to 2 minutes, until set. Repeat with the remaining batter.

Scourge Greek yogurt and maple extract or maple syrup until combined. Serve it over the sweet potato pancakes.

Nutrition: 355 Calories 12g Total Fat 305mg Sodium 477mg Potassium 50g Total Carbohydrate 16g Protein

1 Sweet Potato Pancakes with Maple Yogurt

Preparation Time: 15 minutes

Cooking Time: 20 minutes

Serving: 6

Ingredient:

2 cups whole-wheat flour

1 tablespoon baking powder

1½ teaspoons pumpkin pie spice

½ teaspoon kosher or sea salt

2 tablespoons dark brown sugar

4 tablespoons canola oil

2 large eggs

1 cup sweet potato purée or cooked mashed sweet potato

1½ cups nonfat milk

1 teaspoon pure vanilla extract

Cooking spray

1½ cups plain nonfat Greek yogurt

½ teaspoon maple extract or 1 tablespoon pure maple syrup

Direction

Scourge flour, baking powder, pumpkin pie spice, and salt until combined.

Using a separate mixing bowl, with a hand mixer set on medium speed to beat the brown sugar and canola oil together until fluffy. While the hand mixer is still beating, add one egg at a time until thoroughly combined. Add the sweet potato purée then the milk and vanilla extract until well blended. With a hand mixer to low speed and slowly add the dry ingredient mixture until well blended.

Heat a large nonstick skillet over medium heat. Coat the pan with the cooking spray. Working in batches, ladle ¼-cup dollops of pancake batter into the pan. Cook for 1 to 2 minutes, until bubbles appear on the top, then flip and cook for another 1 to 2 minutes, until set. Repeat with the remaining batter.

Scourge Greek yogurt and maple extract or maple syrup until combined. Serve it over the sweet potato pancakes.

Nutrition: 355 Calories 12g Total Fat 305mg Sodium 477mg Potassium 50g Total Carbohydrate 16g Protein

2 Raspberry Chocolate Scones

Preparation Time: 7 minutes

Cooking Time: 12 minutes

Servings: 2

Ingredients:

1 cup whole-wheat pastry flour

1 cup all-purpose flour

1 tablespoon baking powder

1/4 teaspoon baking soda

1/3 cup trans-fat-free buttery spread

1/2 cup fresh or frozen raspberries

1/4 cup miniature chocolate chips

1 cup plus 2 tablespoons plain fat-free yogurt

2 tablespoons honey

1/2 teaspoon sugar

1/4 teaspoon cinnamon

Directions:

Preheat the oven to 400 degrees F.

Combine flours with baking soda and baking powder in a mixing bowl.

Cut the butter into the dry mixture until it forms a crumbly mixture.

Fold in chocolate chips and berries.

Pour in honey and yogurt, then stir the mixture gently to form a crumbly batter.

Knead the dough ball on a surface then spread it into ½ inch thick circle.

Slice the sheet into 12 wedges, then arrange them on a greased baking tray.

Sprinkle sugar and cinnamon mixture on top.

Bake them for 12 minutes at 400 degrees F.

Serve and enjoy.

Nutrition:

Calories 149

Total Fat 13.7 g

Saturated Fat 12.7 g

Cholesterol 78 mg

Sodium 141 mg

Total Carbs 22.9 g

Fiber 3.2 g

Sugar 1.3 g

Protein 4.2 g

3 Banana Almond Smoothie

Preparation Time: 3 minutes

Cooking Time: 0 minutes

Servings: 2

Ingredients:

10 Ounces (2 large) banana, frozen

4 Tablespoons flaxseeds

2 Tablespoons almond butter

1 Cup almond milk

½ Teaspoon honey

¼ Teaspoon vanilla extract

Directions:

Using a blender, combine all the Ingredients, until it becomes smooth.

Transfer the entire mix into two serving glass.

Serve fresh or refrigerate and consume.

Nutrition:

Calories: 581

Total Fat: 42.5 g

Saturated Fat: 26.8 g

Total carbs: 47.5 g

Dietary Fiber 11.7 g

Total Sugar: 23.8 g

Cholesterol: 0 mg

Sodium: 25 mg

Protein: 10.3 g

Calcium: 35 mg

Iron: 9 mg

Potassium: 1059 mg

Vitamin D: 0 mcg

4 Blueberry Banana Muffins

Preparation Time: 20 minutes

Cooking Time: 25 minutes

Serving: 2

Ingredients:

20 Ounces (4 large) ripe banana, mashed

1¼ Cups blueberries, fresh or frozen

¾ Cup+2 tablespoons almond milk, unsweetened

¼ Cup maple syrup

1 Teaspoon apple cider vinegar

1 Teaspoon vanilla extract

2 Cups white flour

¼ Cup coconut oil

2 Teaspoons baking powder

6 Tablespoons cane sugar

1½ Teaspoons cinnamon, ground

½ Teaspoon baking soda

½ Teaspoon salt

½ Cup walnut halves, chopped

Directions:

Set the oven to 360°F and preheat.

Spray some cooking oil into the muffin tin.

In a standard-sized bowl, mash all bananas and take ¾ cup.

The remaining portion refrigerates for making the smoothie.

Put the mashed banana into a bowl along with the vinegar, milk, maple syrup, and vanilla. Do not stir.

In a big bowl, mix all the dry Ingredients like sugar, flour, cinnamon, baking powder, salt, and baking soda.

Stir in coconut oil into the dry mixture and combine well.

Pour all wet items mentioned in step 4 on top of the dry Ingredients and blend it. Avoid over mixing.

Put walnuts into the mix and after that the blueberries, and make sure that you have not over mix the Ingredients. Over mixing may make it like a thick batter and the muffin become strong and spoil the dish.

Spoon ¼ cup of batter into every tin of muffin,

Bake the muffin at 370°F for 22 to 27 minutes.

Insert a toothpick to check it baking status. When inserted the toothpick, it should come out clean.

After baking is over, keep it 5-8 minutes to settle down and transfer to the cooling rack, keep it there for 15 minutes.

Serve fresh.

Nutrition:

Calories: 296

Total Carbohydrates: 36.3 g

Dietary Fiber: 1.7 g

Sugars: 16.4 g

Total Fat: 14.6 g

Saturated Fat: 9.5 g

Cholesterol: 0 mg

Sodium: 161 mg

Protein: 3.9 g

5 Easy Buckwheat Crepes

Preparation Time: 10 minutes

Cooking Time: 15 minutes

Serving: 2

Ingredients:

For making Crepes:

1 Cup buckwheat flour, raw, un-toasted

1¾ Cups light coconut milk, low-fat

¾ Tablespoon flaxseed

1 Tablespoon melted coconut oil

⅛ Teaspoon ground cinnamon

⅛ Teaspoon salt

⅛ Teaspoon stevia

For fillings:

8 Tablespoons nut butter

6 Tablespoons granola

6 Tablespoons compote

8 Tablespoons -coconut whipped cream

3 Cinnamon baked apples

Directions:

Put buckwheat flour, flaxseed, light coconut milk, coconut oil, salt, cinnamon and stevia into a blender.

Blend the above Ingredients until it combines well. Blend until it turns into a pourable batter. Add a little buckwheat flour if the dough is too thin. If the batter is too thick, add some dairy-free milk.

Heat a nonstick skillet on medium temperature. Once, the skillet is hot, spread some oil in the bottom evenly.

When the oiled surface of skillet becomes hot, pour ¼ cup of batter into the skillet and cook until the top turns bubbly and the edges become dry. Carefully flip the crepes to cook for 2 minutes more. Do not let the skillet become too hot.

Repeat the process until you finish all the crepes. To keep the warmness of the crepes, keep parchment paper between the crepes.

Serve it with the vegan butter, or maple syrup or nut butter, or coconut whipped cream or cinnamon banked apples. You can also serve it with bananas or berries.

Best if you serve it fresh, but you can easily store leftovers sealed in the refrigerator up to 3 days. You can use it after reheating.

Nutrition:

Calories: 230

Total Fat: 16.6 g

Saturated Fat: 8.1 g

Total Carbs: 24.6 g

Dietary Fiber: 3.2 g

Total Sugars: 3 g

Cholesterol: 0 mg

Sodium: 39 mg

Protein: 4.2 g

6 Peanut Butter Oats in the Jar

Preparation Time: 6 hours and 5 minutes

Cooking Time: 0 minutes

Servings: 1

Ingredients

For the oats:

½ cup gluten-free rolled oats

½ cup unsweetened, plain almond milk

4 tablespoons natural salted peanut butter

1 tablespoon maple syrup (or stevia, organic brown sugar)

¾ tablespoon chia seeds

For the toppings (optional):

Banana, sliced

Strawberries or raspberries

Chia seeds

Directions:

Combine the almond milk, peanut butter, chia seeds, and maple syrup in a Mason jar. Stir but don't over-mix to leave swirls of peanut butter. Add the oats and stir again.

Press down the oats with a spoon to make sure they are soaked in the milk mixture.

Secure the jar with a lid and refrigerate for at least 6 hours.

To serve, garnish with toppings of choice.

Note: Nutritional info does not include toppings.

Nutrition:

Calories: 454

Carbohydrates: 50.9g

Fat: 3.9g

Saturated Fat: 2g

Fiber: 12g

Protein: 14.6g

Sodium: 162mg

Sugar: 14.9g

7 Fruit Smoothie

Preparation Time: 5 minutes

Cooking Time: 5 minutes

Servings: 1

Ingredients:

One-fourth cup blueberries

Four oz. strawberries

One-half orange, peeled

Four oz. papaya peeled, seeded and diced

One-fourth cup ice cubes

Four oz. soy milk

Directions:

Pulse the blueberries, strawberries, peeled orange, and milk in a blender for approximately half a minute.

Combine the ice cubes and papaya and continue to blend for another 30 seconds.

Transfer to a glass and enjoy immediately.

You can also use frozen fruit if you prefer.

Nutrition:

Sodium: 71 mg

Protein: 6 g

Fat: 3 g

Sugar: 26 g

Calories: 184

Soup

8 Loving Cauliflower Soup

Preparation time: 15 minutes

Cooking time: 10 minutes

Servings: 6

Ingredients:

4 cups vegetable stock

1-pound cauliflower, trimmed and chopped

7 ounces Kite ricotta/cashew cheese

4 ounces almond butter

Sunflower seeds and pepper to taste

Directions:

Put almond butter and melt in a skillet over medium heat.

Add cauliflower and sauté for 2 minutes. Add stock and bring the mix to a boil.

Cook until cauliflower is al dente. Stir in cream cheese, sunflower seeds, and pepper. Puree the mix using an immersion blender. Serve and enjoy!

Nutrition: Calories: 143

Fat: 16g Carbohydrates: 6g Protein: 3.4g Sodium: 510 mg

9 Garlic and Lemon Soup

Preparation time: 15 minutes

Cooking time: 0 minutes

Servings: 3

Ingredients:

1 avocado, pitted and chopped

1 cucumber, chopped

2 bunches spinach

1 ½ cups watermelon, chopped

1 bunch cilantro, roughly chopped

Juice from 2 lemons

½ cup coconut aminos

½ cup lime juice

Directions:

Add cucumber, avocado to your blender, and pulse well. Add cilantro, spinach, and watermelon and blend. Add lemon, lime juice, and coconut amino. Pulse a few more times. Transfer to a soup bowl and enjoy!

Nutrition: Calories: 100 Fat: 7g Carbohydrates: 6g Protein: 3g Sodium: 0 mg

10   Cucumber Soup

Preparation time: 15 minutes

Cooking time: 0 minutes

Servings: 4

Ingredients:

2 tablespoons garlic, minced

4 cups English cucumbers, peeled and diced

½ cup onions, diced

1 tablespoon lemon juice

1 ½ cups vegetable broth

½ teaspoon sunflower seeds

¼ teaspoon red pepper flakes

¼ cup parsley, diced

½ cup Greek yogurt, plain

Directions:

Put the listed fixing in a blender and blend to emulsify (keep aside ½ cup of chopped cucumbers). Blend until smooth. Divide the soup amongst 4 servings and top with extra cucumbers. Enjoy chilled!

Nutrition: Calories: 371

Fat: 36g Carbohydrates: 8g Protein: 4g Sodium: 40 mg

11   Roasted Garlic Soup

Preparation time: 15 minutes

Cooking time: 60 minutes

Servings: 10

Ingredients:

1 tablespoon olive oil

2 bulbs garlic, peeled

3 shallots, chopped

1 large head cauliflower, chopped

6 cups vegetable broth

Sunflower seeds and pepper to taste

Directions:

Warm your oven to 400 degrees F. Slice ¼ inch top of the garlic bulb and place it in aluminum foil. Oiled it using olive oil and roast in the oven for 35 minutes. Squeeze flesh out of the roasted garlic.

Heat-up oil in a saucepan and add shallots, sauté for 6 minutes. Add garlic and remaining ingredients. Adjust heat to low. Let it cook for 15-20 minutes.

Puree the mixture using an immersion blender. Season soup with sunflower seeds and pepper. Serve and enjoy!

Nutrition: Calories: 142 Fat: 8g Carbohydrates: 3.4g Protein: 4g Sodium: 548 mg

---

Meat

12   Pork Chops with Thyme and Apples

Preparation time: 10 minutes

Cooking time: 35 minutes

Servings: 4

Ingredients:

1 and ½ cups red onion, cut into wedges

2 and ½ teaspoons olive oil

2 cups apple, cored and cut into wedges

Black pepper to the taste

2 teaspoons thyme, chopped

4 medium pork loin chops, bone-in

1 teaspoon cider vinegar

½ cup low-sodium chicken stock

Directions:

Heat up a pan with 1 teaspoon oil over medium-high heat, add the onions, stir and cook them for 2 minutes.

Add apples, stock, vinegar, black pepper and the thyme, toss introduce the pan in the oven at 400 degrees F and bake for 15 minutes.

Heat up another pan with the rest of the oil over medium-high heat, add pork, season with pepper and cook for 5 minutes on each side.

Add the apples and thyme mix, toss, everything, cook for 5 minutes more, divide between plates and serve.

Nutrition: calories 240, fat 7, fiber 2, carbs 10, protein 17

13   Pork and Roasted Tomatoes Mix

Preparation time: 10 minutes

Cooking time: 15 minutes

Servings: 6

Ingredients:

1 pound pork meat, ground

2 cups zucchinis, chopped

½ cup yellow onion, chopped

Black pepper to the taste

15 ounces canned roasted tomatoes, no-salt-added and chopped

¾ cup low-fat cheddar cheese, shredded

Directions:

Heat up a pan over medium-high heat, add pork, onion, black pepper and zucchini, stir and cook for 7 minutes.

Add roasted tomatoes, stir, bring to a boil, cook over medium heat for 8 minutes, divide into bowls, sprinkle cheddar on top and serve.

Enjoy!

Nutrition: calories 270, fat 5, fiber 3, carbs 10, protein 12

14　　　Pork, Water Chestnuts And Cabbage Salad

Preparation time: 10 minutes

Cooking time: 0 minutes

Servings: 10

Ingredients:

1 green cabbage head, shredded

1 and ½ cups brown rice, already cooked

2 cups pork roast, already cooked and shredded

10 ounces peas

8 ounces water chestnuts, drained and sliced

½ cup low-fat sour cream

½ cup avocado mayonnaise

A pinch of black pepper

Directions:

In a bowl, combine the cabbage with the rice, shredded meat, peas, chestnuts, sour cream, mayo and black pepper, toss and serve cold.

Enjoy!

Nutrition: calories 310, fat 5, fiber 4, carbs 11, protein 17

15   Pork and Zucchini Stew

Preparation time: 10 minutes

Cooking time: 1 hour

Servings: 4

Ingredients:

1 pound round pork, cubed

Black pepper to the taste

¼ teaspoon sweet paprika

1 tablespoon olive oil

1 and ½ cups low-sodium veggie stock

3 cups zucchinis, cubed

1 yellow onion, chopped

½ cup low-sodium tomato sauce

1 tablespoon parsley, chopped

Directions:

Heat up a pot with the oil over medium-high heat, add the pork, black pepper and paprika, stir and brown for 5 minutes. Add stock, onion and tomato sauce, toss, bring to a simmer, reduce heat to medium and cook for 40 minutes.

Add the zucchinis and the parsley, toss, cook for 15 minutes more, divide into bowls and serve.

Enjoy!

Nutrition: calories 270, fat 7, fiber 9, carbs 12, protein 17

16   Pork Roast, Leeks and Carrots

Preparation time: 10 minutes

Cooking time: 1 hour and 10 minutes

Servings: 4

Ingredients:

2 pounds pork roast, trimmed

4 carrots, chopped

4 leeks, chopped

1 teaspoon black peppercorns

2 yellow onions, cut into wedges

1 tablespoon parsley, chopped

1 cup low-sodium veggie stock

1 teaspoon mustard

Black pepper to the taste

Directions:

Put the pork in a roasting pan, add carrots, leeks, peppercorns, onions, stock, mustard and black pepper, toss, cover the pan and bake in the oven at 375 degrees F for 1 hour and 10 minutes.

Slice the meat, divide it between plates, sprinkle parsley on top and serve with the carrots and leeks mix on the side. Enjoy!

Nutrition: calories 260, fat 5, fiber 7, carbs 12, protein 20

Seafood

17   Spring Salmon Mix

Preparation time: 10 minutes

Cooking time: 0 minutes

Servings: 4

Ingredients:

2 tablespoons scallions, chopped

2 tablespoons sweet onion, chopped

1 and ½ teaspoons lime juice

1 tablespoon chives, minced

1 tablespoon olive oil

1 pound smoked salmon, flaked

1 cup cherry tomatoes, halved

Black pepper to the taste

1 tablespoon parsley, chopped

Directions:

In a bowl, mix the scallions with sweet onion, lime juice, chives, oil, salmon, tomatoes, black pepper and parsley, toss and serve.

Enjoy!

Nutrition: calories 200, fat 8, fiber 3, carbs 8, protein 6

18   Smoked Salmon and Green Beans

Preparation time: 10 minutes

Cooking time: 0 minutes

Servings: 4

Ingredients:

3 tablespoons balsamic vinegar

2 tablespoons olive oil

1/3 cup kalamata olives, pitted and minced

1 garlic clove, minced

Black pepper to the taste

½ teaspoon lemon zest, grated

1 pound green beans, blanched and halved

½ pound cherry tomatoes, halved

½ fennel bulb, sliced

½ red onion, sliced

2 cups baby arugula

¾ pound smoked salmon, flaked

Directions:

In a bowl, combine the green beans with cherry tomatoes, fennel, onion, arugula and salmon and toss.

Add vinegar, oil, olives, garlic, black pepper and lemon zest, toss and serve.

Enjoy!

Nutrition: calories 212, fat 3, fiber 3, carbs 6, protein 4

19   Saffron Shrimp

Preparation time: 10 minutes

Cooking time: 30 minutes

Servings: 4

Ingredients:

1 teaspoon lemon juice

Black pepper to the taste

½ cup avocado mayo

½ teaspoon sweet paprika

3 tablespoons olive oil

1 fennel bulb, chopped

1 yellow onion, chopped

2 garlic cloves, minced

1 cup canned tomatoes, no-salt-added and chopped

1 and ½ pounds big shrimp, peeled and deveined

¼ teaspoon saffron powder

Directions:

In a bowl, combine the garlic with lemon juice, black pepper, mayo and paprika and whisk.

Add the shrimp and toss.

Heat up a pan with the oil over medium-high heat, add the shrimp, fennel, onion and garlic mix, toss and cook for 4 minutes.

Add tomatoes and saffron, toss, divide into bowls and serve.

Enjoy!

Nutrition: calories 210, fat 2, fiber 5, carbs 8, protein 4

20   Crab, Zucchini And Watermelon Soup

Preparation time: 4 hours

Cooking time: 0 minutes

Servings: 4

Ingredients:

¼ cup basil, chopped

2 pounds tomatoes

5 cups watermelon, cubed

¼ cup red wine vinegar

1/3 cup olive oil

2 garlic cloves, minced

1 zucchini, chopped

Black pepper to the taste

1 cup crabmeat

Directions:

In your food processor, mix tomatoes with basil, vinegar, 4 cups watermelon, garlic, 1/3 cup oil and black pepper to the taste, pulse, pour into a bowl and keep in the fridge for 1 hour. Divide this into bowls, add zucchini, crab and the rest of the watermelon and serve.

Enjoy!

Nutrition: calories 231, fat 3, fiber 3, carbs 6, protein 8

Vegetarian and Vegan

21   Tofu Parmigiana

Preparation Time: 15 minutes

Cooking Time: 8 minutes

Servings: 2

Ingredients:

6 oz firm tofu, roughly sliced

1 teaspoon coconut oil

1 teaspoon tomato sauce

½ teaspoon Italian seasonings

Directions:

In the mixing bowl, mix up, tomato sauce, and Italian seasonings.

Then brush the sliced tofu with the tomato mixture well and leave for 10 minutes to marinate.

Heat up coconut oil.

Then put the sliced tofu in the hot oil and roast it for 3 minutes per side or until tofu is golden brown.

Nutrition:

83 calories,

7g protein,

1.7g carbohydrates,

6.2g fat,

0.8 fiber,

1mg cholesterol,

24mg sodium,

135mg potassium.

22 Mushroom Stroganoff

Preparation Time: 10 minutes

Cooking Time: 20 minutes

Servings: 2

Ingredients:

2 cups mushrooms, sliced

1 teaspoon whole-grain wheat flour

1 tablespoon coconut oil

1 onion, chopped

1 teaspoon dried thyme

 1 garlic clove, diced

1 teaspoon ground black pepper

½ cup of soy milk

Directions:

Heat up coconut oil in the saucepan.

Add mushrooms and onion and cook them for 10 minutes.

Stir the vegetables from time to time.

After this, sprinkle them with ground black pepper, thyme, and garlic.

Add soy milk and bring the mixture to boil.

Then add flour and stir it well until homogenous.

Cook the mushroom stroganoff until it thickens.

Nutrition:

70 calories,

2.6g protein,

6.9g carbohydrates,

4.1g fat,

1.5g fiber,

0mg cholesterol,

19mg sodium,

202mg potassium.

23   Eggplant Croquettes

Preparation Time: 15 minutes

Cooking Time: 5 minutes

Servings: 2

Ingredients:

1 eggplant, peeled, boiled

2 potatoes, mashed

2 tablespoons almond meal

1 teaspoon chili pepper

1 tablespoon coconut oil

1 tablespoon olive oil

¼ teaspoon ground nutmeg

Directions:

Blend the eggplant until smooth.

Then mix it up with mashed potato, chili pepper, coconut oil, and ground nutmeg.

Make the croquettes from the eggplant mixture.

Heat up olive oil in the skillet.

Put the croquettes in the hot oil and cook them for 2 minutes per side or until they are light brown.

Nutrition:

180 calories,

3.6g protein,

24.3g carbohydrates,

8.8g fat,

7.1g fiber,

0mg cholesterol,

9mg sodium,

721mg potassium.

24   Stuffed Portobello

Preparation Time: 10 minutes

Cooking Time: 20 minutes

Servings: 2

Ingredients:

4 Portobello mushroom caps

½ zucchini, grated

1 tomato, diced

1 teaspoon olive oil

½ teaspoon dried parsley

¼ teaspoon minced garlic

Directions:

In the mixing bowl, mix up diced tomato, grated zucchini, dried parsley, and minced garlic.

Then fill the mushroom caps with zucchini mixture and transfer in the lined with baking paper tray.

Bake the vegetables for 20 minutes or until they are soft.

Nutrition:

24 calories,

1.2g protein,

2.9g carbohydrates,

1.3g fat,

0.9g fiber,

0mg cholesterol,

5mg sodium,

238mg potassium.

25   Chile Rellenos

Preparation Time: 10 minutes

Cooking Time: 30 minutes

Servings: 2

Ingredients:

2 chili peppers

2 oz vegan Mozzarella cheese, shredded

 2 oz tomato puree

1 tablespoon coconut oil

 2 tablespoons whole-grain wheat flour

1 tablespoon potato starch

¼ cup of water

½ teaspoon chili flakes

Directions:

Bake the chili peppers for 15 minutes in the preheated to 375F oven.

Meanwhile, pour tomato puree in the saucepan.

Add chili flakes and bring the mixture to boil. Remove it from the heat.

After this, mix up potato starch, flour, and water.

When the chili peppers are cooked, make the cuts in them and remove the seeds.

Then fill the peppers with shredded cheese and secure the cuts with toothpicks.

Heat up coconut oil in the skillet.

Dip the chili peppers in the flour mixture and roast in the coconut oil until they are golden brown.

Sprinkle the cooked chilies with tomato puree mixture.

Nutrition:

187 calories,

4.2g protein,

16g carbohydrates,

12g fat,

3.7g fiber,

0mg cholesterol,

122mg sodium,

41mg potassium.

Side Dishes, Salads & Appetizers

26 Greek Salad

Preparation time: 6 minutes

Cooking Time: Nil

Serving: 4

Ingredients:

2 cucumbers, diced

2 tomatoes, slice

1 green lettuce, cut into thin strips

2 red bell peppers, cut

½ cup black olives pitted

3 ½ ounces feta cheese, cut

1 red onion, sliced

2 tablespoons olive oil

2 tablespoons lemon juice

Sunflower seeds and pepper to taste

Direction

Dice cucumbers and slice up the tomatoes.

Tear the lettuce and cut it into thin strips.

De-seed and cut the peppers into strips.

Take a salad bowl and mix in all the listed vegetables, add olives and feta cheese (cut into cubes).

Take a small cup and mix in olive oil and lemon juice, season with sunflower seeds and pepper.

Pour mixture into the salad and toss well, enjoy!

Nutrition:

Calories: 132

Fat: 4g

Carbohydrates: 3g

Protein: 5g

27   Fancy Greek Orzo Salad

Preparation time: 5 minutes and 24 hours chill time

Cooking Time: 10 minutes

Serving: 4

Ingredients:

1 cup orzo pasta, uncooked

½ cup fresh parsley, minced

6 teaspoons olive oil

1 onion, chopped

1 ½ teaspoons oregano

Directions:

Cook the orzo and drain them.

Add to a serving dish.

Add 2 teaspoons of oil.

Take another dish and add parsley, onion, remaining oil and oregano.

Season with sunflower seeds, pepper according to your taste.

Pour the mixture over the orzo and let it chill for 24 hours.

Serve and enjoy at lunch!

Nutrition:

Calories: 399

Fat: 12g

Carbohydrates: 55g

Protein:16g

28   Homely Tuscan Tuna Salad

Preparation time: 5-10 minutes

Cooking Time: Nil

Serving: 4

Ingredients:

15 ounces small white beans

6 ounces drained chunks of light tuna

10 cherry tomatoes, quartered

4 scallions, trimmed and sliced

2 tablespoons lemon juice

Directions:

Add all of the listed ingredients to a bowl and gently stir.

Season with sunflower seeds and pepper accordingly, enjoy!

Nutrition:

Calories: 322

Fat: 8g

Carbohydrates: 32g

Protein:30g

29   Asparagus Loaded Lobster Salad

Preparation time: 10 minutes

Cooking Time: Nil

Serving: 4

Ingredients:

8 ounces lobster, cooked and chopped

3 ½ cups asparagus, chopped and steamed

2 tablespoons lemon juice

4 teaspoons extra virgin olive oil

¼ teaspoon kosher sunflower seeds

Pepper

½ cup cherry tomatoes halved

1 basil leaf, chopped

2 tablespoons red onion, diced

Directions:

Whisk in lemon juice, sunflower seeds, pepper in a bowl and mix with oil.

Take a bowl and add the rest of the ingredients.

Toss well and pour dressing on top.

Serve and enjoy!

Nutrition:

Calories: 247

Fat: 10g

Carbohydrates: 14g

Protein: 27g

30 Supreme Spinach and Mushroom Lasagna

Preparation time: 10 minutes

Cooking time: 40 minutes

Servings: 2

Ingredients:

1 tablespoon of olive oil

1 medium sized diced onion

4 minced garlic cloves

8 ounces of white mushroom diced

3 cups of frozen chopped spinach

1 teaspoon of red pepper flakes

9 no-boil oven ready lasagna sheets

1 - ½ cup of marinara sauce

1 – ½ cup of vegan cheese

½ a cup of cashew cream

Directions:

Set your pot to Sauté mode and add oil, garlic and cook for 2 minutes

Add mushrooms, spinach and red pepper flakes

Cook for 2 minutes

Take the veggies out and keep them on a plate

Rinse your pot well and add cashew cream and vegan cheese on another bowl

Break your pasta sheets and arrange them evenly in the cake pan

Spread ½ cup of sauce on top

Spread half of the spinach and mushroom on top

Spread half of the cheese on top

Place spaghetti sheet and keep repeating the whole process until all the ingredients are used up

Place a trivet in your Instant Pot

Cover the cake pan with foil and place the pan on top of the trivet

Seal the lid and cook at HIGH pressure for 10 minutes

Release the pressure naturally

Nutrition: 380 Calories 14g Fat 48g Carbohydrates 17g Protein 217mg Potassium 106mg Sodium

31   Uber Cauliflower and Potato Mash

Preparation time: 5 minutes

Cooking time: 15 minutes

Servings: 2

Ingredients:

1 and a ½ cups of water

2 pounds of potatoes sliced up into 1-inch pieces

8 ounce of cauliflower florets

½ a teaspoon of flavored vinegar

1 minced garlic clove

Directions:

Add water to your Instant Pot

Add potatoes and sprinkle cauliflower florets on top

Close and cook at HIGH pressure for 5 minutes

Release the pressure naturally over 10 minutes

Sprinkle a bit of flavored vinegar and garlic

Mash and serve!

Nutrition: 249 Calories 0.6g Fat 55g Carbohydrates 7.5g Protein 251mg Potassium 113mg Sodium

32   Satisfying Corn Cob

Preparation time: 5 minutes

Cooking time: 11 minutes

Servings: 2

Ingredients:

8 ears of corn

2 cups of water

Directions:

Husk the corns and cut the bottom part of the corns, wash them well thoroughly

Wash well

Add water to the cooker base and arrange the corns vertically with the large part submerged underwater and the small part pointing upward

Cover and cook at HIGH pressure for 2 minutes

Release the pressure naturally

Serve with a bit of flavored vinegar and vegan butter

Nutrition: 63 Calories 1g Fat 14g Carbohydrates 2.4 Protein 241mg Potassium 110mg Sodium

33   Multi-Purpose Mushroom and Pate Spread

Preparation time: 15 minutes

Cooking time: 15 minutes

Servings: 2

Ingredients:

¾ cup of porcini mushroom

1 cup of water

1 tablespoon of olive oil

1 tablespoon of coconut oil

1 sliced shallot

1 pound of white button mushroom

¼ cup of white wine vinegar

1 and a ½ teaspoon of flavored vinegar

½ a teaspoon of white pepper

1 piece of bay leaf

1 tablespoon of truffle oil

3 tablespoons of grated vegan cheese

Directions:

Add porcini mushroom to a heat proof measuring cup. Pour boiling water over the mushroom

Cover and keep it on the side

Set your pot to Sauté mode and add olive and coconut oil, allow the oil to heat up

Add shallots and Sauté for a while. Add fresh mushroom and Sauté until golden

Pour wine vinegar and allow it to evaporate

Add porcini mushroom and liquid, pepper, flavored vinegar and bay leaf

Seal and cook at HIGH pressure for 12 minutes. Perform quick release. Discard the bay leaf and add olive oil. Puree the mixture using an immersion blender and enjoy!

Nutrition: 63 Calories 1g Fat 14g Carbohydrates 2.4g Protein 241mg Potassium 104mg Sodium

34   Borders Apart Mexican Cauliflower Rice

Preparation time: 5 minutes

Cooking time: 5 minutes

Servings: 2

Ingredients:

6 cups of brown rice (cooked)

1 can of fire roasted tomatoes

2 cups of salsa

4 tablespoon of tomato paste

3 cups of chopped onion

6 cloves of garlic

1 and a ½ cups of water

Directions:

Add the listed ingredients to your Instant Pot.

Close and cook at HIGH pressure for 5 minutes. Release the

pressure naturally

Stir in chopped cilantro and top up with your desired

toppings. Enjoy!

Nutrition: 562 Calories 25g Fat 63g Carbohydrates 23g Protein

101mg Potassium 84mg Sodium

35   Resourceful Potato Salad

Preparation time: 10 minutes

Cooking time: 15 minutes

Servings: 2

Ingredients:

2 pound of potato cut up into bite sized portions

2 cups of water

1 cup of diced carrots

1 cup of green peas

1 can of chickpeas

For Sauce

2 tablespoon of olive oil

1 and a ½ teaspoon of cumin seeds

1 teaspoon of coriander seeds

½ a teaspoon of mustard seeds

1 and a ½ teaspoon of Garam masala

1 teaspoon of minced garlic

Cilantro and Chutney ingredients

½ a cup of packed mint leaves

½ a cup of packed fresh cilantro

½ an inch knob of fresh ginger cut up into pieces

¼ cup of water

2 teaspoon of lime juice

½ a teaspoon of flavored vinegar

Directions:

Add carrots, potato and water to your Instant Pot

Close and cook at HIGH pressure for 10 minutes and release the pressure naturally

Add peas and lock the lid

Lock up the lid and cook for a few seconds at low pressure

Remove the lid and give it a few minutes

Pour the mixture into a colander and rinse with cold water

Take a pan and add oil over medium heat

Add oil and heat it up, add coriander seeds, cumin seeds and mustard seeds

Sauté them for about 2 minutes until they release a nice fragrance

Lower down the heat and add Garam Masala alongside minced garlic

Sauté for 1 minute more

Remove the heat and allow it to cool

Add the listed ingredients under "Cilantro and Chutney" and to a food processor and pulse until you have a smooth texture

Situate a big sized mixing bowl and mix in cooked veggies, the cooled up Sautéed oil/spice mi and chutney

Add the chickpeas and mix well

Chill for an hour if you want and enjoy!

Nutrition: 440 Calories 27g Fat 46g Carbohydrates 6g Protein 191mg Potassium 64mg Sodium

---

Dessert and Snacks

36   Tasty Mediterranean Peanut Almond butter Popcorns

Preparation time: 5 minutes + 20 minutes chill time

Cooking Time: 2-3 minutes

Serving: 4

Ingredients:

3 cups Medjool dates, chopped

12 ounces brewed coffee

1 cup pecans, chopped

½ cup coconut, shredded

½ cup cocoa powder

Directions:

Soak dates in warm coffee for 5 minutes.

Remove dates from coffee and mash them, making a fine smooth mixture.

Stir in remaining ingredients (except cocoa powder) and form small balls out of the mixture.

Coat with cocoa powder, serve and enjoy!

Nutrition:

Calories: 265

Fat: 12g

Carbohydrates: 43g

Protein 3g

37   Just A Minute Worth Muffin

Preparation time: 5 minutes

Cooking Time: 1 minutes

Serving: 2

 Ingredients:

Coconut oil for grease

2 teaspoons coconut flour

1 pinch baking soda

1 pinch sunflower seeds

1 whole egg

Directions:

Grease ramekin dish with coconut oil and keep it on the side.

Add ingredients to a bowl and combine until no lumps.

Pour batter into ramekin.

Microwave for 1 minute on HIGH.

Slice in half and serve.

Enjoy!

Nutrition:

Total Carbs: 5.4

Fiber: 2g

Protein[MOU5]: 7.3g

38   Hearty Almond Bread

Preparation time: 15 minutes

Cooking Time: 60 minutes

Serving: 8

Ingredients:

3 cups almond flour

1 teaspoon baking soda

2 teaspoons baking powder

¼ teaspoon sunflower seeds

¼ cup almond milk

½ cup + 2 tablespoons olive oil

3 whole eggs

Directions:

Preheat your oven to 300 degrees F.

Take a 9x5 inch loaf pan and grease, keep it on the side.

Add listed ingredients to a bowl and pour the batter into the loaf pan.

Bake for 60 minutes.

Once baked, remove from oven and let it cool.

Slice and serve!

Nutrition:

Calories: 277

Fat: 21g

Carbohydrates: 7g

Protein: 10g

39   Mixed Berries Smoothie

Preparation time: 4 minutes

Cooking Time: 0 minutes

Serving: 2

Ingredients:

¼ cup frozen blueberries

¼ cup frozen blackberries

1 cup unsweetened almond milk

1 teaspoon vanilla bean extract

3 teaspoons flaxseeds

1 scoop chilled Greek yogurt

Stevia as needed

Directions:

Mix everything in a blender and emulsify.

Pulse the mixture four time until you have your desired thickness.

Pour the mixture into a glass and enjoy!

Nutrition:

Calories: 221

Fat: 9g

Protein: 21g

Carbohydrates: 10g

40 Satisfying Berry and Almond Smoothie

Preparation time: 10 minutes

Cooking Time: Nil

Serving: 4

Ingredients:

1 cup blueberries, frozen

1 whole banana

½ cup almond milk

1 tablespoon almond butter

Water as needed

Directions:

Add the listed ingredients to your blender and blend well until you have a smoothie-like texture.

Chill and serve.

Enjoy!

Nutrition:

Calories: 321

Fat: 11g

Carbohydrates: 55g

Protein: 5g

41   Refreshing Mango and Pear Smoothie

Preparation time: 10 minutes

Cooking Time: Nil

Serving: 1

Ingredients:

1 ripe mango, cored and chopped

½ mango, peeled, pitted and chopped

1 cup kale, chopped

½ cup plain Greek yogurt

2 ice cubes

Directions:

Add pear, mango, yogurt, kale, and mango to a blender and puree.

Add ice and blend until you have a smooth texture.

Serve and enjoy!

Nutrition:

Calories: 293

Fat: 8g

Carbohydrates: 53g

Protein: 8g

42   Epic Pineapple Juice

Preparation time: 10 minutes

Cooking Time: Nil

Serving: 4

Ingredients:

4 cups fresh pineapple, chopped

1 pinch sunflower seeds

1 ½ cups water

Directions:

Add the listed ingredients to your blender and blend well
until you have a smoothie-like texture.

Chill and serve.

Enjoy!

Nutrition:

Calories: 82

Fat: 0.2g

Carbohydrates: 21g

Protein: 21

43   Choco Lovers Strawberry Shake

Preparation time: 10 minutes

Serving: 1

Ingredients:

½ cup heavy cream, liquid

1 tablespoons cocoa powder

1 pack stevia

½ cup strawberry, sliced

1 tablespoon coconut flakes, unsweetened

1 ½ cups water

Directions:

Add listed ingredients to blender.

Blend until you have a smooth and creamy texture.

Serve chilled and enjoy!

Nutrition:

Calories: 470

Fat: 46g

Carbohydrates: 15g

Protein: 4g

44   Healthy Coffee Smoothie

Preparation time: 10 minutes

Serving: 1

Ingredients:

1 tablespoon chia seeds

2 cups stongly brewed coffee, chilled

1 ounce Macadamia Nuts

1-2 packets stevia, optional

1 tablespoon MCT oil

Directions:

Add all the listed ingredients to a blender.

Blend on high until smooth and creamy.

Enjoy your smoothie.

Nutrition:

Calories: 395

Fat: 39g

Carbohydrates: 11g

Protein: 5.2g

45   Blackberry and Apple Smoothie

Preparation time: 5 minutes

Serving: 2

Ingredients:

2 cups frozen blackberries

½ cup apple cider

1 apple, cubed

2/3 cup non-fat lemon yogurt

Directions:

Add the listed ingredients to your blender and blend until smooth.

Serve chilled!

Nutrition:

Calories: 200

Fat: 10g

Carbohydrates: 14g

Protein 2g

46   The Mean Green Smoothie

Preparation time: 5 minutes

Serving: 2

Ingredients:

1 avocado

1 handful spinach, chopped

Cucumber, 2 inch slices, peeled

1 lime, chopped

Handful of grapes, chopped

5 dates, stoned and chopped

1 cup apple juice (fresh)

Directions:

Add all the listed ingredients to your blender.

Blend until smooth.

Add a few ice cubes and serve the smoothie.

Enjoy!

Nutrition:

Calories: 200

Fat: 10g

Carbohydrates: 14g

Protein 2g

47   Mint Flavored Pear Smoothie

Preparation time: 5 minutes

Serving: 2

Ingredients:

¼ honey dew

2 green pears, ripe

½ apple, juiced

1 cup ice cubes

½ cup fresh mint leaves

Directions:

Add the listed ingredients to your blender and blend until smooth.

Serve chilled!

Nutrition:

Calories: 200

Fat: 10g

Carbohydrates: 14g

Protein 2g

48   Chilled Watermelon Smoothie

Preparation time: 5 minutes

Serving: 2

Ingredients:

1 cup watermelon chunks

½ cup coconut water

1 ½ teaspoons lime juice

4 mint leaves

4 ice cubes

Directions:

Add the listed ingredients to your blender and blend until smooth.

Serve chilled!

Nutrition:

Calories: 200

Fat: 10g

Carbohydrates: 14g

Protein 2g

49   Banana Ginger Medley

Preparation time: 5 minutes

Serving: 2

Ingredients:

1 banana, sliced

¾ cup vanilla yogurt

1 tablespoon honey

½ teaspoon ginger, grated

Directions:

Add the listed ingredients to your blender and blend until smooth.

Serve chilled!

Nutrition:

Calories: 200

Fat: 10g

Carbohydrates: 14g

Protein 2g

50   Banana and Almond Flax Glass

Preparation time: 5 minutes

Serving: 2

Ingredients:

1 ripe frozen banana, diced

2/3 cup unsweetened almond milk

1/3 cup fat free plain Greek Yogurt

1 ½ tablespoons almond butter

1 tablespoon flaxseed meal

1 teaspoon honey

2-3 drops almond extract

Directions:

Add the listed ingredients to your blender and blend until smooth

Serve chilled!

Nutrition:

Calories: 200

Fat: 10g

Carbohydrates: 14g

Protein 2g

Conclusion

10 Tips For Dash

If you are trying the diet for the first time, I am sure you will be anxious about how to go about it. To put you out of your misery, I have compiled several tips, with respect to the DASH diet, in this chapter.

Getting Started

1. Take it slow: Ensure that the change is gradual. As of now, if you are eating only one or two servings of fruits and vegetables every day, try including one more serving at lunch or dinner. You can increase it to the requisite servings gradually. Similarly, if you are not

used to consuming whole grains, don't try to switch over immediately. Start including whole grains in one or two servings. This will help you avoid bloating and diarrhea, which are commonly associated with the sudden consumption of fiber in large quantities. In order to avoid gas, which is commonly associated with the intake of beans and vegetables, you may also try over the counter products. One rule is to always soak your whole grains and lentils before cooking as that help in reducing your gas and bloating tendencies. You will find it easy to incorporate them in your diet. But again, don't do it all at once. You have to learn to take it slow and remain as patient with your body as possible. It is known that many people give up on the diet just because they are experiencing elevated bouts of diarrhea but if you keep doing that then you will not be able to stick with any diet.

2. Make sure you reward successes: Since this is the first time you will be trying this diet plan, make sure that you have a proper reward system in place. It will not be possible for you to adhere to the diet 100% in the very first week. Make room for these little failures. If you are prepared for these little failures, you will not be discouraged to follow the diet because of a small slip up. On the contrary, if you strive to achieve perfection from the beginning, you will only be disappointed. Disappointment can often discourage you from following a diet plan. When you see that you have deviated from the diet, try to identify the reason behind the slip up. Your job does not end with just identifying the reason. Try to figure out ways to ensure that the

slip up does not happen again. Resume the DASH diet where you left it.

On the other hand, it is necessary that you acknowledge your little successes and reward it wisely. Make sure that the rewards are non-food items. It can be as simple as renting a movie or visiting a friend. When you learn to acknowledge these little successes, you will be motivated to follow the diet. You can also promise someone else something nice as that will help you remain motivated for a long time. The basic idea is to motivate yourself to do something that you think will make you stick with the diet. You can promise your children something nice like a play station and you can use it as a motivation to continue with your diet. Similarly, you should think of something that will force you to remain with your diet and do your best to better it every single time.

3. Physical exercise: The DASH diet, coupled with physical exercise, cannot only help you lower your blood pressure but also help you lose weight easily. Hence, ensure that you spend some time for exercising every day. We looked at the simple exercises that you can try out. Don't worry if you are not an exercising person. Your body will have the capacity to adjust to a new schedule. You only have to put in the right efforts and the results will come through for you. Many people make the mistake of doing too much at the very beginning and then give up on it altogether. That is not the right way to go about it and you have to take it slow at the beginning and then gradually increase the intensity. Remember that what you do today will only show effect tomorrow. Expecting too much at once is never a good idea for anyone.

4. Get external advice: If you are finding it difficult to stick to the diet, do not hesitate to get in touch with a dietician or doctor. They may help you overcome the difficulties you are facing with respect to the diet. You have sit down with them and discuss everything in detail. Give them a clear picture of your body and tell them if you are suffering from any illnesses. Once everything is laid out in front of them, they will be able to give you an appropriate advice.

5. Form a support system: The success of any diet plan depends on your levels of motivation. If you are not motivated, you will not be able to get through the diet at all. As I mentioned before, the DASH diet is a long-term approach. Hence, it is important that your motivation levels are high, if you wish to adopt the DASH diet in the long run. Seek the help of family and friends to meet your diet goals. Keep them briefed about your diet goals and the reason why you want to follow this diet. This way, your friends and family will be in a position to motivate you, when you find it difficult to follow the diet. Also, when you keep them in the loop, the chances of them tempting you into deviating from the diet are very less.

6. Make a list: Plan your meals well ahead. Before you head out for shopping, you should have a clear idea about the dishes you are going to cook over the week. Only if you are clear about the dishes that you are going to cook will you be able to prepare a list of the ingredients that are required. Ensure that you put down every single ingredient in your list. Remember that you will require ingredients for preparing DASH

snacks and breakfasts too. So, do not forget to include them in your list. When you have a list in hand, you will be able to shop better in a focused fashion. Most often, people tend to stray away from the diet and end up shopping processed foods and snacks, mainly because they don't have a proper grocery list on hand. Hence, it all rides on how detailed your grocery list is.

7. Eat before you go shopping: You may wonder how this is a relevant tip. Think about the number of times you have grabbed a snack from the shelves because you were hungry while shopping. This could be an important reason behind you deviating from the diet. When we are hungry, we don't bother checking labels and ingredients. We just grab the snack within our reach to satisfy our hunger. Hence, make sure that you eat well before you go shopping. This way, you will buy only the things mentioned in your grocery list and not consume anything that could possibly make you deviate from your diet. If you think you have the tendency of walking towards the wrong items then you should immediately stop yourself and walk away from it. You can also ask a friend to go with you in order to stop you from going towards the wrong items.

8. Buy Fresh: As you know, the DASH diet discourages the consumption of processed and refined foods because of their sodium and fat content. Hence, the key is to buy fresh ingredients. Fresh foods contain low quantities of sodium, fat and are devoid of added sugar, salt and preservatives. They also have more flavors as opposed to processed foods. Another important reason why fresh foods are better is because

they are packed with fiber, vitamins and minerals. If you are opting for the canned versions of fresh foods, such as canned vegetables, make sure that you pick only those that have reduced fat and sodium.

9. Maintain a journal: Write down everything you eat. This way, you will find it easier to identify the pain points in your diet. For instance, if you are facing bloating issues, it could be because of the sudden inclusion of fibers in your diet. When you look at your journal, you will be able to monitor your intake of fiber in such a fashion that you don't face bloating issues. Another advantage of maintaining a journal is that you will be able to find out if you are allergic to certain kinds of foods. You can choose between a physical journal and a digital journal. The advantage of a digital journal is that it will be available for use on all your devices and you can pull it up at any time. But you will get a unique feel if you use a physical journal and might find it a bit personal to use one. Another reason why having a diet journal is advantageous is because it will help you shop wisely next time. Now that you have a clear idea of how much you eat, what foods you are allergic to, you will be able to pick out the ingredients for your meals in a prudent fashion.

10. Cook your own meals: The best way to ensure that you stick to the diet is by cooking your own meals. When you cook your own meals, you will be able to ensure that all the ingredients that you use and the techniques that you adopt are DASH friendly. If it is possible to make all of your ingredients from scratch, then go for it. For instance, if you are cooking pasta, try to make

your own pasta instead of going for store made pasta. Similarly, make your own sauce instead of opting for readymade sauce.

CPSIA information can be obtained
at www.ICGtesting.com
Printed in the USA
BVHW011010060321
601714BV00027B/150